Anonymus

Outlines of Anatomy

A Guide to the Dissection of the Human Body

Anonymus

Outlines of Anatomy
A Guide to the Dissection of the Human Body

ISBN/EAN: 9783742831781

Manufactured in Europe, USA, Canada, Australia, Japa

Cover: Foto ©Lupo / pixelio.de

Manufactured and distributed by brebook publishing software
(www.brebook.com)

Anonymus

Outlines of Anatomy

A GUIDE

TO THE

DISSECTION OF THE HUMAN BODY

BASED ON GRAY'S ANATOMY

———

GEORGE WAHR
PUBLISHER AND BOOKSELLER
ANN ARBOR, MICH.

PREFACE.

The objects of this outline are to inform the student what structures are found in each region and where the description of each structure is found in Gray's Anatomy. The outline is based on Gray's Anatomy—thirteenth edition, dated 1897. The figures in parentheses refer to the pages and to the plates in Gray's Anatomy.

UPPER DISSECTION.

Cranial Region.

>Surface form of head and face (222).
>
>Outline superficial nerves of head and face (814)
>(Fig. 489).
>
>Outline arteries of head and face (553) (Fig. 349).
>
>Outline veins of head and face (651) (Fig. 381).
>
>*Dissection* (391).
>
>Coverings of skull are: 1. Skin, 2. Superficial fascia,
>3. Occipito-frontalis and its aponeurosis, 4. Loose
>connective tissue, 5. Periosteum.
>
>Skin of scalp (391).
>
>Superficial fascia (392).

NERVES:

>Supra-orbital (798).
>
>Supratrochlear (798).
>
>Auriculo-temporal (806).
>
>Orbital or temporo-malar (801).
>
>Temporal branches of seventh (814).
>
>Occipitalis major (828).
>
>Occipitalis minor (831).

ARTERIES:

>Supra-orbital (568).
>
>Frontal (570).
>
>Superficial temporal (558) (Fig. 349).
>
>Posterior auricular (557).
>
>Occipital (557).

VEINS:

>Supra-orbital (651).
>
>Frontal (651).
>
>Temporal (652).
>
>Posterior auricular (653).
>
>Occipital (653).

Lᴙᴍᴘʜᴀᴛɪᴄꜱ:
 Read lymphatics of head, face and neck (681).
Mᴜꜱᴄʟᴇꜱ:
 Occipito-frontalis (392).

Auricular Region.

 Dissection (393).
Mᴜꜱᴄʟᴇꜱ:
 Attrahens aurem (393).
 Attollens aurem (394).
 Retrahens aurem (394).
Nᴇʀᴠᴇꜱ:
 Posterior auricular (813).
 Auricular branches of auricularis magnus (813).
Aʀᴛᴇʀɪᴇꜱ:
 Posterior auricular (557).

FACE.—(Fig. 26).

External Palpebral and Orbital Region (392) (Fig. 269.)

 The appendages of the eye (907).
 The lachrymal apparatus (909).
 Dissection (394) (Figs. 268–269).
Mᴜꜱᴄʟᴇꜱ:
 Orbicularis palpebrarum (394).
 Corrugator supercilii (395).
 Levator palpebræ superioris (396).
 Tensor tarsi (395).
 Tendo oculi (395).
Nᴇʀᴠᴇꜱ:
 Supra-orbital (798).
 Supratrochlear (798).
 Infratrochlear (799).
Aʀᴛᴇʀɪᴇꜱ:
 Supra-orbital (569),
 Frontal (570).
 Nasal (570).

Palpebral (570).

Lachrymal (568).

Expose the tendons of muscles inserted into sclerotic coat of eye (396) (Fig. 271).

Nasal Region.—(Fig. 269).

MUSCLES OF NOSE (398–399).

Superior, Inferior and Inter-Maxillary Regions. (Fig. 269).

Dissection (394) (Fig. 268).

MUSCLES:

Superior maxillary region (400).

Inferior maxillary (400).

Inter-maxillary (401–402).

Platysma myoides (407) (Fig. 269).

PAROTID GLAND (946) (Fig. 569).

Description of gland (945–946).

NERVES:

Facial (814) (Fig. 487).

Description (811–812–813–814).

Branches:

Temporo-facial { Temporal. Malar. Infra-orbital.

Cervico-facial { Supra-maxillary. Infra-maxillary. Buccal.

Brances of fifth nerve (Fig. 482).

Description (796).

Infraorbital (803).

Malar (801).

Auriculo-temporal (806).

Mental (807).

Mylo-hyoid (807).

Auricularis magnus (831).

ARTERIES: (Fig. 349).
    Facial (554).
    Transverse facial (559) (Fig. 349).
    Middle temporal (559).
    Infra-orbital (562).
    Inferior dental—Mental branches (561).

VEINS: (Fig. 381).
    Frontal (651).
    Supra-orbital (651).
    Angular (651).
    Facial (652).
    Temporal (652).
    Internal maxillary (653).
    Temporo-maxillary (653).
    Posterior auricular (653).

FASCIA:
    Masseteric (403).
    Temporal (403).

Skull.
    Vertex (208),
    Lateral region (214).
    Temporal fossa (215).
    Spheno-maxillary fossa (216).
    Anterior region (217).
    Orbit (217–218–219).

Remove skull-cap as described on p. 702.

Internal surface of skull-cap (208).
    Middle meningeal artery (560).

Membranes of brain.
    Dura mater (703).
    Arachnoid (704).
    Pia mater (705).

Remove brain.

Exit of cranial nerves through dura mater and base of skull.

Veins of diploe (615) (Fig. 382).

The Eye.

Dissect the eye of an ox or sheep.

Dissection (894).

Capsule of Tenon (890).

Tunics.

1. Sclerotic (891) and cornea (892).
2. Choroid (891), iris (896) and ciliary processes (898).
3. Retina (898).

Refracting media.

1. Aqueous humor (903).
2. Vitreous body (903).
3. Crystalline lens and its capsule (904).

The Neck.

Landmarks—Locate: Median line of neck, thyroid cartilage, clavicle and lower jaw, and mastoid process.

Surface form (427).

Outline superficial veins (Fig. 381).

Outline arteries (Figs. 347–352).

Outline nerves (Fig. 489).

Dissection (407).

Superficial structures.

    Superficial fascia (407).

    Platysma myoides (407) (Fig. 269).

    Deep cervical fascia (407) (Fig: 275)).

VEINS: (Fig. 281).

    External jugular and tributaries (653).

    Posterior external jugular (654).

    Anterior jugular (654).

    Study veins of head and neck (650).

NERVES: (Fig. 489).

    Cervical plexus.

        Superficial branches (831).

    Infra-maxillary of facial (815).

    Lymphatic glands of neck (683).

Deeper dissection of neck.

Triangles of the Neck (566).

Posterior Triangles (565).

Study the description of the posterior triangle given on p. 565 before beginning the dissection.

OCCIPITAL AND SUBCLAVIAN TRIANGLES (565).

NERVES:

Cervical plexus and branches (831) (Figs. 496–489–494).

Spinal accessory (823) (Fig. 489–491–492).

MUSCLES: (Figs. 276–285).

Sterno-cleido-mastoid (409).

Omo-hyoid (412).

Trapezius (428).

Scaleni (425) (Figs. 276–284–285).

Splenius capitis (433) (Figs. 276–285).

Levator anguli scapulae (431) (Fig. 276).

ARTERIES: (Fig. 347).

Suprascapular and branches (585) (Fig. 347).

Transversalis colli and branches (585) (Fig. 347).

Third portion of subclavian (578) (Fig. 347).

Anterior Triangles (563) (Fig. 276).

Study the description given on pp. 563 and 564 before beginning the dissection. Study Figs. 276–277–285–345–352–494.

NERVES of inferior and superior carotid triangles (Figs. 494--492).

Hypoglossal and descendens hypoglossi (823) (Fig. 494).

Communicans hypoglossi (833) (Figs. 493–494).

Ansa hypoglossi.

Superior laryngeal (821) (Fig. 492).

Pneumogastric (819) (Figs. 491–492).

Inferior or recurrent laryngeal (821) (Figs. 491–492).

Sympathetic (867–869–871) (Figs. 513–572).

Phrenic (833) (Figs. 494–496).

Review deep branches of cervical plexus (831).

MUSCLES of inferior and superior carotid triangles.

Sterno-mastoid (409).
Omo-hyoid (412).
Sterno-hyoid (411).
Sterno-thyroid (411).
Thyro-hyoid (411).
Scaleni (425).

ARTERIES of inferior and superior carotid triangles.
(Fig. 347).

Common carotid (547).
External carotid (551).
Superior thyroid (552).
Lingual (553) (Fig. 352).
Ascending pharyngeal (558) (Fig. 352).
Facial (554) (Figs. 347-349-352).
Occipital (556) (Figs. 347-349).
Posterior auricular (557) (Figs. 347-349).
Subclavian (576-7-8) (Figs. 347-352-359-360).
Thyroid axis (584) (Fig. 347).
Branches of thyroid axis (584-585) (Figs. 347-361).
Vertebral (581) (Fig. 352).
Branches (582).
Internal mammary (586) (Fig. 360).
Superior intercostal (587) (Fig. 352).

VEINS OF NECK (653) (Figs. 381-386).
Internal jugular (654).
Tributaries to internal jugular (654-655).
Subclavian (665).
Tributaries to subclavian (665) (Fig. 388).

THORACIC DUCT (680) (Fig. 394).

LYMPHATIC GLANDS (683) (Figs. 395-6).
Superficial and deep (683).

THYROID GLAND (1122).

THYMUS GLAND (1124).

Submaxillary Triangle (564) (Figs. 276-277-347-352).
Superficial structures *only.*

MUSCLES:
Digastric (413).
Stylo-hyoid (413).
Mylo-hyoid (413).

ARTERIES: Facial (554).

NERVES: Hypoglossal (823) (Fig. 494).

SUBMAXILLARY GLAND (947) (Fig. 569).
Do not remove this gland now.

Temporo- and Pterygo-Maxillary Regions. (Figs. 273 and 274).
Masseter fascia and muscle (403).
Temporal fascia (403).
Dissection (403).
Temporal muscle (403) (Fig. 273).

MUSCLES OF MASTICATION: (493).
Masseter (404).
Temporal (403).
Dissection (404).
External pterygoid (404) (Fig. 274).
Internal pterygoid (405) (Fig. 274).

ARTERIES: (Figs. 350-351).
Internal maxillary and branches (559-560-561-562).

VEINS:
Internal maxillary (652).

TEMPORO-MAXILLARY ARTICULATION (327).
Ligaments (327-328-329) (Figs. 232-233-234).
Action (329).

NERVES:
Inferior maxillary of fifth and branches (805-806-807) (Figs. 482-483).
Otic ganglion (807) (Fig. 485).
Chorda tympani (812) (Fig. 483).

Branches of seventh at its exit (812).
    Digastric (813).
    Stylo-hyoid (813).
    Posterior auricular (813).
LYMPHATICS of head (681) (Figs. 395–396).

Submaxillary Triangle—Deep Structures.

Submaxillary gland (947) (Figs. 569).
Submaxillary ganglion (808) (Fig. 482–483).
MUSCLES:
    Mylo-hyoid (414) (Fig. 277).
    Hyo-glossus (416) (Fig. 278).
    Genio-hyoid (414) (Figs. 277–278).
    Genio-hyo-glossus (415) (Fig. 278).
    Stylo-glossus (416) (Fig. 278).
    Stylo-pharyngeus (419) (Fig. 282).
NERVES:
    Hypoglossal (823) (Figs 493–494).
    Lingual (807) (Fig. 483).
    Inferior dental (807) (Figs. 482–350).
        Mylo-hyoid (807).
    Chorda tympani (812) (Fig. 483).
ARTERIES:
    Lingual and branches (553) (Fig. 352).
    Inferior dental (561) (Fig. 350).
    Facial—cervical portion (554).
VEINS:
    Lingual (554).
LYMPHATICS (683) (Fig. 395–396).
SUBLINGUAL GLAND (948) (Fig. 569).

Deep Dissction of the Neck.

STYLO-PHARYNGEUS MUSCLE (419).
GLOSSO-PHARYNGEAL NERVE (816) (Figs. 490–491–492).
INTERNAL CAROTID ARTERY (565) (Figs. 347–352).
ASCENDING PHARYNGEAL ARTERY (558) (Fig. 352).
    L UVENJNGULAR VEIN (654) (Fig. 386).

PNEUMOGASTRIC NERVE (819) (Figs. 491–492).

HYPOGLOSSAL NERVE (823).

GANGLIATED CORD AND CERVICAL GANGLIA OF SYM-
PATHETIC (869) (Figs. 512–513).

Anterior Vertebral Region.

*Remove the anterior part of the skull with the pharynx
attached by dividing the trachea, oesophagus and other
structures about one inch below the larynx. Draw the
trachea and oesophagus forward and separate them
from their anterior vertebral attachment. At base of
skull divide basilar process of occipital bone with a
chisel. With a saw cut inward along the posterior
border of petrous portion of temporal bone, passing
behind the jugular foramen and join the cut made with
the chisel. Wrap the part removed in a wet cloth and
lay aside while the anterior vertebral region is being
dissected.*

Dissection of Anterior Vertebral Region.

MUSCLES: (Fig. 284).

Longus colli (425).

Rectus capitis anticus major (424).

Rectus capitis anticus minor (424).

Rectus capitis lateralis (425).

Scaleni on lateral vertebral region (425) (Fig. 284).

ARTERIES:

Vertebral and branches (581–2–3) (Fig. 352).

Profunda cervicis (587) (Fig. 352).

VEINS:

Vertebral and tributaries (655).

NERVES:

Trunks of the cervical and brachial plexuses are
exposed.

Deep branches of cervical plexus (333).

ARTICULATIONS:

Atlas with axis (323–324).
Atlas with occipital (325–6).
Axis with occipital (326–7).

Pharynx.

Examine mouth, palate, tonsil, uvula, pillars of fauces, openings of Eustachian tubes and nares (Fig. 552).
Description of pharynx (951).
MUSCLES: (Figs. 282–283).
Inferior constrictor (419).
Middle constrictor (420).
Superior constrictor (420).
Stylo-pharyngeus (420).
Palato-pharyngeus (422).
Salpingo-pharyngeus (423).
Open the pharynx by a median incision through its posterior wall.

Mouth.

DESCRIPTION OF MOUTH (930–1).

Palate.

DESCRIPTION OF PALATE (944–5).
MUSCLES: (Fig. 283).
Levator palati (421).
Tensor palati (422).
Azygos uvulæ (422).
Palato-glossus (422).
Palato-pharyngeus (422).

Tonsils.

DESCRIPTION: (945).

Tongue (Fig. 515).

DESCRIPTION (879–880–881–2–3).

MUSCLES (Figs. 278–279–280–519–520).

> Extrinsic:
>> Genio-hyo-glossus (415).
>> Hyo-glossus (416).
>> Stylo-glossus (416).
>> Palato-glossus (416).
>> Chondro-glossus (416).
> Intrinsic:
>> Description (pp. 416–417–1418).

Larynx (1100).

> DESCRIPTION (pp. 1101 to 1108 inclusive).

> *Dissection: Cut the thyroid cartilage a little to one side of anterior median line and turn the smaller piece off to expose the muscles attached to arytenoid cartilage.*

Supra-Maxillary Region.

> *Expose the superior maxilary division of fifth nerve by cutting the bones to outer side of spheno-maxilary fissure and infra-orbital groove.*

> SUPERIOR MAXILLARY NERVE AND BRANCHES (801) (Figs. 482–483–484).

> SPHENO-PALATINE OR MECKEL'S GANGLION (803) (Figs. 483–484).

> INTERNAL MAXILLARY ARTERY.
>> Branches of spheno-maxillary portion (562) (Figs 352–351).

Nose.

> *Open nasal cavity by a vertical incision just to one side of median line.*

> Description of nose (835–886).
> Description of nasal fossæ (219–2220–221–222) (886–887–888–889).
> Surgical anatomy (889–890).

The Back.

LANDMARKS:
    Vertebral spines.
    Surface form (440).
    Dissection (428) (Fig. 286).
SUPERFICIAL AND DEEP FASCIA (428).
MUSCLES:
    First layer (428) (Fig. 287).
    Second layer (431) (Fig. 287).
    Third layer (432) (Fig. 287).
    Vertebral aponeurosis (433).
    Lumbar fascia (433) (Figs. 287-295,.
    Fourth layer (434) (Fig. 288).
    Fifth layer (437) (Fig. 288).
    Suboccipital triangle (439) (Fig. 288).
NERVES:
    Cervical, posterior division (828) (Figs. 495-502).
    Dorsal, posterior division (845) (Fig. 502).
    Lumbar, posterior division (849) (Fig. 502).
    Sacral, posterior division (857) (Fig. 507).
    Coccygeal, posterior division (858).
    Spinal accessory (823) (Fig. 492).
ARTERIES:
    Intercostal (606).
        Anterior branches (607).
        Posterior branches (608).

Pectoral and Axillary Regions.

LANDMARKS: Clavicle, sternum, mammary gland, ribs, axilla (587-8-9), scapula and its processes, and shoulder joint.
    Outline heart (1086) (Fig. 694).
    Dissection (Fig. 301).
    Superficial fascia (466).
    Deep fascia (466).
    Mammary gland (1178).

MUSCLES:

Pectoralis major (467) (Fig. 302).

Dissection (467).

Costo-coracoid membrane (468).

Pectoralis minor (469) (Fig. 303).

Subclavius (469) (Fig. 303).

Deltoid (471) (Fig. 302).

Deep fascia (471).

Serratus magnus (470) (Fig. 303-4).

Fascia (471).

Subscapular fascia (472).

Subscapular (472) (Fig. 303).

Dissection (473).

Supraspinous fascia (473).

Supraspinatus (473) (Fig. 305).

Infraspinous fascia (473).

Infraspinatus (473) (Fig. 305).

Teres major (474) (Fig. 305).

Teres minor (474) (Fig. 305).

ARTERIES OF PECTORAL REGION.

Perforating of internal mammary (586).

Branches of axillary (589) (Fig. 362).

ARTERIES OF AXILLA.

Axillary and its branches (589-590-1-2-3) (Fig. 362).

Study subclavian artery and branches (576-577-578-579-580).

VEINS:

Axillary and branches (664).

Subclavian and branches (665).

NERVES:

Pectoral region.

Anterior thoracic (838) (Fig. 500).

Dorsal, anterior division (846).

First dorsal (846).

Upper dorsal and branches (846-7-8).

Axillary nerves:
Brachial plexus (834–5–6–7–8) (Figs. 497–500).
LYMPHATICS (684–5–6).

Thorax and Thoracic Viscera.

LANDMARKS: Ribs, sternum and clavical.
*Cut the cartilages where they join the ribs and remove
them with the sternum.* Note˙ internal mammary
artery and branches (586).
THORAX (1083).
Cavity.
Upper opening.
Lower opening.
MUSCLES:
Intercostal fascia (441).
Intercostal muscles (441) (Fig. 303).
External (442).
Internal (442).
Infracostalis (442).
Triangularis sterni (442) (Fig. 289).
Levatores costarum (442) (Fig. 283).
Muscles of inspiration and expiration (444).
Diaphragm (444–5–6–7) (Fig. 290).
PERICARDIUM (1082–3–3–5) (Figs. 692–3).
PLEURA (1113–4) (Fig. 707).
MEDIASTINUM (1114–5–6).
Study the position and relation of heart and large
blood vessels, trachea and lungs (Figs. 344–5–6–388–
394–694–707–710–711).
THE HEART: (1086–7–8–9–1090–1–2–3–4–5).
FOETAL PECULIARITIES IN VASCULAR SYSTEM (1096).
FOETAL CIRCULATION (1097–8–9).
ARTERIES: (539).
Pulmonary (540) (Fig. 344).

Aorta (541) (Fig. 344).
Ascending aorta (541).
Arch of aorta (543-4).
Coronary (542-3) (Fig. 344).
Branches of arch of aorta (545) (Figs. 344-345).
Innominate (545).
Thyroidea ima (545).
Descending aorta (605).
Thoracic aorta and its branches (605-6-7-8)
(Fig. 708).
Superior intercostal (587) (Fig. 352).
Internal mammary and branches (586).

NERVES.

Phrenic (833).
Pneumogastric (819-20-1-2).
Dorsal:
First dorsal (846).
Upper dorsal and branches (846-7).
Thoracic gangliated cord (872-3).

VEINS:

Innominate right and left (665) (Fig. 388).
Internal mammary (666).
Inferior thyroid (666) (Fig. 388).
Superior intercostal (666) (Fig. 388).
Superior vena cava (667) (Fig. 388).
Azygos and tributaries (667) (Fig. 388).
Spinal veins (668-9) (Fig. 389-90).

LYMPHATICS:

Thoracic duct (680-1) (Fig. 394).
Lymphatics of thorax (691-2).

SURGICAL ANATOMY OF THE UPPER EXTREMITY (499-
500-501-502).

ARTICULATIONS OF RIBS WITH VERTEBRÆ (330-1-2-3)
(Figs. 235-236).

2

ARTICULATIONS OF CARTILAGES OF RIBS WITH STERNUM (333–4) (Fig. 238).

ARTICULATIONS OF CARTILAGES WITH EACH OTHER (334–5) (Fig. 238).

ARTICULATIONS OF RIBS WITH THEIR CARTILAGES (335) (Fig. 238).

LIGAMENTS OF STERNUM (336).

Arm and Forearm.

LANDMARKS:

Bones of elbow joint.

Outline arteries and veins and superficial lymphatics, and nerves of arm and forearm (363–364–365–387–498–499–500–397).

Dissection (475).

FASCIA (475).

MUSCLES OF ARM:—

Anterior:

Coraco-brachialis (476) (Figs. 302–3).

Biceps (476) (Figs. 302–3).

Brachialis anticus (477) (Figs. 302–3).

Posterior:

Triceps (477) (Fig. 305).

Subanconeus (478).

Latissimus dorsi (430) (Figs. 287–305).

MUSCLES OF FOREARM:

Dissection (478–481–483).

Fascia (478).

Anterior radio-ulnar region.

Superficial layer (479–80–81) (Fig. 306).

Fibrous sheaths (481).

Deep layer (481–2–3) (Fig. 307).

Radial region (483–4–5) (Fig. 308).

Posterior radio-ulnar region.

Superficial layer (485–6) (Fig. 308).

Deep layer (486–7–8–9) Fig. 310).

NERVES OF ARM.

Brachial plexus (834) (Fig. 497).

Cutaneous branches (Figs. 498–499).

Branches: (Figs. 497–500–401).

Suprascapular (837) (Fig. 501).

Subscapular (838).

Circumflex (839) (Fig. 501).

External and internal thoracic (838).

Lesser internal cutaneous (840).

Internal cutaneous (839).

Ulnar (841).

Musculo-spiral (842).

Median (840).

Musculo-cutaneous (839).

NERVES OF FOREARM.

Cutaneous (Fig. 498–499).

Circumflex (839) (Fig. 501).

Internal cutaneous (839).

Ulnar (841).

Median (840).

Musculo-spiral and its branches (842–843–844).

Radial and posterior interosseous (844).

ARTERIES OF ARM.

Brachial and its branches (593–4–5–6) (Fig. 363).

ARTERIES OF FOREARM.

Radial and its branches (597–8–9) (Fig. 364–365).

Ulnar and its branches (601–2–3–4) (Fig. 364–5–6).

VEINS OF ARM AND FOREARM (462–3–4) (Fig. 387).

LYMPHATICS (684–5–6) (Fig, 397).

Wrist and Hand.

LANDMARKS:

Bony points. Palmar arches (604).

Dissection (489).

Anterior annular ligament (489) (Fig. 311).

Synovial membrane of flexor tendons (480) (Fig. 312).

Posterior annular ligament (490).
Deep palmar fascia (490–1–2) (Fig. 314).
Superficial transverse ligament of fingers (492).
MUSCLES:
    Of the thumb (492–3–4) (Figs. 315–316).
    Of the little finger (494–5–6) (Fig. 316).
    Palmaris brevis (494) (Fig. 316).
    Middle palmar (496–7) (Figs. 317–318).
NERVES:
    Median (840) (Fig. 500).
    Ulnar (841) (Fig. 500).
    Radial (844) (Fig. 499).
    Interosseus anterior (841).
    Interosseus posterior (844) (Fig. 501).
ARTERIES:
    Radial and branches at wrist (598–9–0).
    Radial and branches at hand (598–9–0–1).
    Ulnar and branches at wrist (601–2–3–4).
    Ulnar and branches at hand (602–3–4).
VEINS:
    Of upper extremity (662).

Articulations (313).

    Bone (313).
    Cartilage)313).
    Ligaments (313).
    Synovial membrane (313).
        Bursal (314),
        Vaginal (314).
    Synovia (314).
ARTICULATION OF UPPER EXTREMITY (340).
    Sterno-clavicular (340–1–2) (Fig. 242).
    Acromio-clavicular (342–3–4) (Fig. 243).
    Ligaments of scapula (344–5) (Fig. 243).
    Shoulder-joint (345–6–7–8) (Fig. 243–4).
    Elbow-joint (349–0–1–2) (Fig. 245–6–7).

Radio-ulnar (353–4–5–6) (Fig. 245-6–8).
Radio-carpal, or wrist-joint (356–7) (Figs. 248–9).
Carpal (357–8–9) (Figs. 248-9).
Carpo-metacarpal (359–0–1).
Metacarpo-phalangeal (361–2) (Fig. 252).
Phalangeal (362) (Fig. 255).
Blood supply and nerve supply of the above articulations.

LOWER DISSECTION.

The Abdomen.

LANDMARKS: Umbilicus, linea alba (455), semilunaris
(456), Poupart's ligament (450), external abdominal
ring (449), internal abdominal ring (456), inguinal
canal (457), crest of ilium (275), anterior superior
spine of ilium (275), anterior inferior spine (275),
os pubis and its spine, crest and angle (277). Lower
ribs, ensiform appendix (229).
(Read pp. 955–956–957–958–959.)

The Abdominal Cavity and Contents. (959).

Regions (959–960–961) (Fig. 578).
How divided (Fig. 578).
Right hypochondrium.
Epigastrium.
Left hypochondrium.
Right lumbar.
Umbilical.
Left lumbar.
Right iliac.
Pubic.
Left iliac.
Give contents of each region (p. 962).
Study Fig. 579—giving posterior view.

Abdominal Walls.

Dissection (447) (Fig. 292).
Superficial fascia (447).
External oblique muscle (448) (Fig. 291).
Aponeurosis of external oblique (448).
Relations (448), Petit's triangle (449).

External abdominal ring (449) (Fig. 757).
Intercolumnar fibers and fascia (450) (Fig. 757).
Poupart's ligament (450) Fig. 292).
Gimbernat's ligament (450).
Triangular ligament (451) (Fig. 758).
Before detaching the external oblique muscles study the surgical anatomy of hernia found on pp. 1180–1181– 1182–1183.
Dissection (451).
Internal oblique (451) (Fig. 293).
Conjoined tendon (452) (Fig. 759–0).
Aponeurosis (452).
Cremaster muscle (452) (Fig. 293).
Cremaster fascia (452).
Dissection (453).
Transversalis muscle (453) (Fig. 294).
Study the surgical anatomy of hernia given on pp. 1184–· 1185–1186.
Dissection (453).
Rectus abdominis (453) (Fig. 294–295).
Lineæ transversæ (456).
Semi-lunar fold of Douglas (455).
Sheath of rectus (454) (Fig. 295).
Pyramidalis (455).
Linea alba (455).
Lineæ semilunares (456).
Transversalis fascia (456).
Internal abdominal ring (456).
Inguinal canal (457).
Deep crural arch (457).
NERVES:
Lower dorsal (848).
Last dorsal (848).
Of lumbar plexus:
Ilio-hypogastric (851) (Fig. 504).
Ilio-inguinal (851) (Fig. 504).

ARTERIES:
From femoral (Fig. 376):
Superficial epigastric (635).
" circumflex iliac (635).
" external pudic (635).
From external iliac (Fig. 372).
Deep epigastric (629).
" circumflex iliac (630).
From internal mammary:
Superior epigastric (587).
From intercostal (606):
Lower intercostals (608).
From lumbar (617):
Abdominal branches (617).
LYMPHATICS:
Superficial lymphatics of the walls of abdomen (689)
(Fig. 398).
Superficial inguinal glands (686).
Review the surgical anatomy of hernia on pp. 1181–2–3–4–5–6.

Inguinal Hernia.

Definition of hernia (1186).
Varieties (1186):
OBLIQUE INGUINAL HERNIA (1187).
Description (1187).
Coverings (1187).
Seat of stricture (1188).
Congenital (1189).
Infantile and encysted (1189).
Funicular process (1189).
DIRECT HERNIA (1189).
Description (1189–0–1).
Hesselbach's triangle (1190).
Coverings (1191).
Seat of stricture (1191).

Spermatic Cord (1155).

  Description (1155).

    Structure (1155).

Contents of Abdomen.

  Open the abdominal cavity as described under Peritoneum, pages 962-3.

  Study description on pages 963-4-5.

  Notice the urachus (113, 963, 1443) (Fig 581).

  Notice the obliterated hypogastric artery (621, 1099) (Fig. 698, 581).

  Notice the umbilical vein (1099) (Fig. 998).

  Study the contents of each region of abdomen in place (962), the position of each organ and their relations to each other and surrounding parts. Note the position the different organs occupy to landmarks.

  POSITION AND RELATIONS OF STOMACH (1001–1003) (Fig. 636). FIXATION OF STOMACH (1003).

  RELATIONS OF DUODENUM (1014–5–6–7).

  MEANS OF FIXATION OF DUODENUM (1018).

  RELATIONS OF LARGE INTESTINES:

    Cæcum (1036).

    Vermiform appendix (1032–3) Fig. 652).

    Ascending colon (1037).

    Transverse colon (1037).

    Descending colon (1037).

    Sigmoid colon (1037).

    Rectum (1043).

  RELATIONS OF LIVER (1055–6).

  FIXATION OF LIVER (1056).

  RELATIONS OF GALL-BLADDER (1064).

  RELATIONS OF SPLEEN (1076) (Fig. 687).

  FIXATION OF SPLEEN (1076).

  RELATIONS OF PANCREAS (1071) (Fig. 634, 584).

The Peritoneum (962).

Adult Peritoneum (978).

Omenta (991).

Great omentum (991).

Lesser omentum (991–2).

Foramen of Winslow (992).

Lesser sac or bursa omentalis (993).

Retro-peritoneal fossæ (994).

Duodenal fossæ (994–5).

Fossa intersigmoidea (996).

Pericæcal fossæ (997).

Dissection.

Expose the structures between the layers of peritoneum forming the mesentery and meso-colon. Work out and expose as far as possible without destruction of the parts and before any of the organs are removed the following structures:

Superior mesenteric artery and its branches (412–3–4) (Figs. 370–1).

Coeliac axis and branches (610–1–2) (Figs. 368–9).

Inferior mesenteric artery and branches (614–5) (Fig. 371).

Portal system of veins (675–6–7) (Fig. 393).

Ducts:—Hepatic, cystic and common bile (1063–4) (Figs. 368–677).

Study and work out as far as possible the sympathetic plexuses described on pp. 875–6–7 (Figs. 512–14).

Remove Jejunum and Ileum.

To do this tie two ligatures around the jejunum at its beginning and divide the intestine between the ligatures. Divide the ileum in same manner several inches above its termination. Divide the mesentery near the intestines. Wash out and study the part removed.

Jejunum and ileum (1020).

Structure of walls (1020).

Serous coat (1020).

Muscular coat (1020).

Submucous coat (1020).
Mucous membrane (1021).
Valvulæ conniventes (1021).
Villi (1022).
Intestinal true glands:
Glands of Lieberkühn (1024).
Glands of Brunner (1024).
Intestinal lymph-follicles:
Solitary glands (1025).
Peyer's patches (1025).
ARTERIES of jejunum and ileum (1026).
Superior mesenteric (612) (Fig. 370).
VEINS (1027): See portal system (675) (Fig. 393).
LYMPHATICS (1027).
NERVES (1027).

Remove Large Intestine.

Ligate the large intestine above the brim of pelvis and divide it. Remove by cutting fixation structures of colon and great omentum along the lower border of stomach below the gastro-epiploic arteries. Wash out and study the part removed. The first part of colon, cæcum and remaining part of ileum should be inflated and allowed to dry, then study ileo-cæcal valve and appendix.

Large intestines (1027–8).
Names of the different parts (1028).
Structure of the large intestine (1028).
Serous coat (1028).
Muscular coat (1028).
Submucous coat (1029).
Mucous membrane (1029).
Crypts of Lieberkühn (1029).
Solitary glands (1029).
ARTERIES:
Superior mesenteric (612).
Ileo-colic (614).
Colica dextra (614).
Colica media (614).

Inferior mesenteric (614).

Colica sinistra (614):

Sigmoidea (614).

VEINS:

Portal system (675) (Fig. 393).

LYMPHATICS (1029).

NERVES (1030).

CÆCUM.

Description, pp. 1030-1-2.

VERMIFORM APPENDIX.

Description, pp. 1032-3.

ILEO-COLIC or ILEO-CÆCAL VALVE.

Description, pp. 1033-4 (Figs. 653-4-5).

COLON (1035):

Ascending colon (1035).

Transverse colon (1035).

Descending colon (1035-6).

Sigmoid flexure (1036).

Expose the coeliac axis and its branches (610) (Figs. 368-369).

Branches of coeliac axis:

Gastric (611) (Fig. 369).

Hepatic and branches (611) (Figs. 368-9).

Splenic and branches (611-12) (Figs. 368-9).

VEINS:

Portal system (675) (Fig. 393).

SYMPATHETIC NERVES:

Solar plexus (875) (Figs. 512-514).

Coeliac plexus (876-7).

Remove the Stomach.

Apply a ligature and divide the œsophagus below the diaphragm. Apply a ligature and divide the duodenum at its beginning. Remove the stomach.

Stomach (999).

Form and size (999-1000) (Figs. 623-4).

Position and relations (1001-2-3).

Points of fixation (1003–4).

Alterations in position (1004).

Structure:

    Serous coat (1004).

    Muscular coat (1004).

    Submucous coat (1005).

    Mucous membrane (1005–6).

        Structure of mucous membrane (1006–7).

ARTERIES (1007):

    Hepatic (611) (Figs. 368–9).

        Pyloric.

        Gastro-epiploica dextra.

    Gastric (611) (Fig. 369).

    Splenic (611) (Figs. 368–9).

        Gastro-epiploica sinistra.

        Vasa brevia.

VEINS (1007).

NERVES (1007).

Inflate duodenum in position and study its relation to pancreas, pancreatic duct, common bile duct, kidneys, superior mesenteric artery and veins; notice parts of duodenum (1014) (Fig. 634).

Study pancreas in place (1067) (Figs. 634–679).

Remove Duodenum and Pancreas.

Duodenum (1008–9).

    Course in adult (1009–10–1).

Peritoneal relations (1081–2–3).

Relations (1014–5–6).

Fixation (1018–9).

ARTERIES:

    Pyloric (611).

    Sup. pancreatico-duodenal (611).

    Inf.   "   "   (613).

NERVES (1026–7).

Pancreas (1067).

    Color.

Volume.

Parts:

Head.

Lesser head.

Body and tail.

Surfaces and borders.

Ducts.

Relations.

Structure (1072).

ARTERIES:

Splenic branches (611).

Pancreatico-duodenalis superior (611).

Pancreatico-dnodenalis inferior (613).

LYMPHATICS (1072).

NERVES (1072).

Remove the Spleen.

Spleen (1073).

Number of spleens (1073).

Volume.

Form and relations (1074–5–6).

Fixation (1076–7).

Position in respiration (1077).

Structure (1077–8–9–0–1).

ARTERIES: Splenic (611).

VEINS: Splenic (675).

LYMPHATICS (1077).

NERVES (1072).

The Liver (1047).

Study the position and relations of the liver in place.

Relations (1055).

Fixation (1056).

Remove the Liver.

Liver—description (1047).

Volume (1047).

Color (1047).
Surfaces (1048–9–10–11).
Fissures (1051).
Lobes (1052).
Ligaments (1053-4).
Peritoneal lines (1054).
ARTERY: Hepatic (1057–611) (Fig. 368).
VEINS: Portal (1057–676) (Fig. 393).
NERVES (1058):
Vagus.
Coeliac plexus.
Structure (1059).
Ducts (1062–3).
Hepatic (1063).
Gall-bladder (1064).
Cystic duct (1064).
Cystic artery (1064).
Cystic veins (1064).
NERVES: Coeliac plexus (1064).
Structure (1065).
Ductus choledochus (1064).

Kidneys and Suprarenal Body.

Expose the kidney and suprarenal body by removing the tissuo in front of them. Study them in place, noting the blood vesels, ureters, and surrounding parts.

Remove ONE kidney with its ureter, cutting ureter at brim of pelvis. Do not remove the other kidney at.this dissection.

Kidney (1127):
Surface form (1135).
Position and size (1127),
Surfaces, borders, and extremities (1127).
Structure of kidney (1128–9).
ARTERIES:
Renal (1133–616) (Fig. 367).

Structures on the Posterior Wall of Abdominal Cavity.

ARTERIES (Figs. 367–388):
Aorta and its branches (608).
 Phrenic (616).
 Coeliac axis (610).
  Gastric.
  Hepatic.
  Splenic.
 Superior mesenteric (612).
 Suprarenal (615).
 Spermatic (616).
 (Ovarian) (616).
 Inferior mesenteric (614).
 Lumbar (617).
 Sacra media (617).
 Common iliac (618) (Fig. 372).
VEINS (Fig. 388):
Inferior vena cava (673).
 Lumbar (674).
 Right spermatic (674).
 (Ovarian) (674).
 Renal (675).
 Suprarenal (675).
 Phrenic (675).
 Hepatic (675).
Portal system (675-6-7) (Fig. 393).
 Review portal system.
Azygos veins (667).
 Tributaries (667).
LYMPHATICS.
Study lymphatics of pelvis and abdomen (687-8-9-0.)
 Of intestines (691).
Thoracic duct (680-1) (Fig. 394).
Deep muscles of abdomen:
 Iliac fascia (503–4).
 Psoas magnus (504) (Fig. 326).
 Psoas parvus (504).

Iliacus (504–5).

Surgical anatomy (505).

Fascia of quadratus lumborum (458).

Quadratus lumborum (458) (Fig. 288).

Lumbar Plexus (850) (Figs. 503–504).

Expose the branches of lumbar plexus by dissecting away carefully part of the psoas magnus muscle. Trace the nerves to their exit from the abdominal cavity.

Branches of lumbar plexus:

Ilio-hypogastric (851).

Ilio-inguinal (851).

Genito-crural (852).

External cutaneous (853).

Anterior crural (855).

Obturator (854).

Accessory obturator (854).

LAST DORSAL NERVE (848).

Pelvic Region.

Study the position and relations of the pelvic organs in place.

Bladder: ·

Position (1138).

Surfaces and peritoneal covering (1140–1–2).

Urachus (1140).

Obliterated hypogastric arteries (1141).

Ligaments (1142–3).

Serous coat (1143).

Vas deferens (1159).

Surface form (1144).

Rectum:

Position.

Relations (1043).

Insert finger into rectum and feel prostate gland.

In female:

Uterus (1168).

Position.

Parts (1168).

Ligaments (1169).

Douglas's pouch (1169).

Appendages of uterus:

    Fallopian tubes (1174) (Fig. 752).

    Ovaries (1175) (Figs. 752–3).

      Ligament of ovary (1175).

Serous covering (1176).

ARTERIES AND VEINS:

Iliac arteries and veins (Fig. 372).

    External and internal (625, 620, 672).

    Division of internal iliac (621).

    Trace visceral branches of internal iliac to where they enter viscera.

    Superior vesical (622).

    Middle   "

    Inferior   "

    Middle hemorrhoidal.·

    Obturator.

SYMPATHETIC NERVES:

Hypogastric plexus (877) (Fig. 512).

Pelvic plexus (878).

Gangliated cord, pelvic portion (874).

Sacral plexus may be exposed.

Ischio-Rectal Region and Perinæum.

Dissection (1201).

Description (1201).

Ischio-rectal region (1201).

Dissection (1201).

Superficial fascia (1201).

MUSCLES:

Corrugator cutis ani (458).

External sphincter (458).

Internal   "   (459).

Levator ani (459) (Figs. 296–771).

Coccygeus (460).

Ischio-rectal fossa (1202).

NERVES.

    Fourth sacral (858).

    Pudic (861).

    Superficial perineal (861).

    Inferior hemorrhoidal (861).

ARTERIES:

    Internal pudic—male and female (624–625).

        Alcock's canal (1202).

        Superficial perineal (625).

        Inferior hemorrhoidal (625).

Perineum in Male.

Description (1202–3).

    Superficial fascia (460).

        Colles' fascia (460) (Fig. 297).

    Deeper perineal fascia or triangular ligament (463–1204–5) (Fig. 769).

        Superficial layer (463).

        Deep layer (463).

        Structures between the two layers (463).

    Central tendinous point (460).

MUSCLES (Fig. 298):

    Accelerator urinæ (461).

    Erector penis (462).

    Transversus perinei (461).

    Compressor urethræ (464).

ARTERIES:

    Internal pudic (623) (Fig. 374).

        Superficial perineal (625).

        Transverse perineal (625).

        Artery of bulb (625).

        Artery of corpus cavernosum (625).

        Dorsal artery of penis (625).

NERVES:

    Pudic and its branches (861–2).

    Inferior pudendal (862).

Cowper's gland (1205-1150).

Position of viscera at outlet of pelvis (1206).

Prostate gland (1206) (Fig. 770).

Surgical anatomy (1207).

Female Perineum (1207).

Description (1207-8).

MUSCLES (464-5).

ARTERIES (625).

NERVES:

Pudic and its branches (861-2).

Remove the pelvic organs. Draw penis down and separate it from pubic arch. Divide levator and sphincter ani muscles. The remaining kidney and ureter should be removed with bladder.

MALE GENERATIVE ORGANS.

Penis (1150).

Description (1150) (Fig. 735).

Structure (1151).

Corpora cavernosa (1151).

Structure (1151-2).

Corpus spongiosum (1152).

Structure (1153).

ARTERIES (625).

LYMPHATICS (1153).

NERVES (1153).

Prostate Gland (1148).

Position, size and form (1148).

Lobes (1149).

Structure (1149).

Nerves and vessels (1149).

Surgical anatomy (1149-0).

Cowper's Gland (1150).

Position and size (1150).

Structure (1150).

Hæmorrhoidal plexus (672).
Common iliac (673).
Middle sacral (673).
Study lymphatics of pelvis (687–8–9–0–1).
Expose sacral plexus (Fig. 508).
Formation (859).
Branches (859).
Exit from pelvis.
SYMPATHETIC NERVES:
Pelvic portion of gangliated cord (874).
Pelvic plexus (878).
Lower Extremity.
LANDMARKS: Poupart's ligament, Scarpa's triangle (630), saphenous opening (Fig. 762), line of femoral artery (Fig. 376).

THIGH.

Anterior Femoral Region.
Dissection (505).
SUPERFICIAL FASCIA.
SUPERFICIAL NERVES (Fig. 506).
Anterior crural:
Middle cutaneous (855).
Internal cutaneous (855).
Muscular (855).
External cutaneous (853) (Figs. 505–6).
Crural branch of genito-crural (852).
Ilio-inguinal (851).
SUPERFICIAL VEINS (Figs. 391–762).
Long saphenous (870).
Superficial epigastric.
"   circumflex iliac.
"   external pudic.
SUPERFICIAL ARTERIES (Fig. 376).
Superficial epigastric (635).
"   circumflex iliac (635).

Superficial external pudic (635).

Superficial inguinal lymphatic glands (686) (Fig. 398).

Femoral Hernia (1191).

Superficial fascia and veins, arteries, nerves and lymphatics contained in it (1191–2–3).

Deep fascia or fascia lata (506–1193).

    Iliac portion.

    Pubic portion.

    Saphenous opening (1194).

Poupart's ligament or crural arch (1195).

Gimbernat's ligament (1196).

Crural Sheath (1196).

Deep crural arch (1197).

Crural canal (1197).

Femoral or crural ring (1198).

Septum crurale (1198).

Descent of hernia (1199).

Coverings of hernia (1199).

Varieties of femoral hernia (1199).

Dissection of Anterior Femoral Region continued:

    Remove fascia lata:

    MUSCLES (Fig. 326):

       Sartorius (508).

       Tensor vaginæ femoris (508).

       Rectus (509).

       Vastus externus (509).

       Vastus internus (510).

       Crureus (510).

       Subcrureus (510).

       Quadriceps extensor (509).

    ARTERIES (Fig. 376):

       Femoral (630):

          Common femoral (631).

            Superficial epigastric (635).

                "   circumflex iliac.

                "   external pudic.

Deep external pudic.

Muscular (637).

Scarpa's triangle (630).

Hunter's canal (630).

Profunda femoris:

Branches will be exposed in dissection of inner thigh.

VEINS (Fig. 391).

Superficial veins have been studied.

Deep veins:

Femoral (672).

NERVES.

Superficial nerves have been studied.

Anterior crural.

Posterior division (855).

Long saphenous (856).

Muscular (856).

Articular (856).

Internal Femoral Region.

Dissection (511).

MUSCLES (Fig. 327).

Gracilis (511).

Pectineus (511).

Adductor longus (512).

"   brevis (512).

"   magnus (513).

ARTERIES:

Profunda femoris.

External circumflex (636).

Internal   "   (636).

Three perforating (636).

Anastomatica magna (637).

Deep external pudic (635).

Obturator (622).

NERVES:

Obturator (854).

Contents (637).

Position of contained parts (637–8).

Popliteal artery (638).

Posterior Femoral Region (Fig. 329).

Dissection (518):

CUTANEOUS NERVES (Fig. 509).

MUSCLES:

Biceps (518).

Semitendinosus (519).

Semimembranosus (519).

NERVES:

Great sciatic (862).

Small sciatic (862).

Obturator (854).

ARTERIES:

Perforating (636).

Popliteal (637).

Branches (639–0–1) (Fig. 377).

The Leg.

LANDMARKS: Study bony projections of knee, ankle and and foot. Examine figures 377–378–391–392–398–505–506–509–510.

Study deep fascia of leg.

Dissection of anterior tibio-fibular region and dorsum of foot (520–1).

Fascia of leg (520), of foot (530).

Anterior annular ligament (528).

Internal	"	"	(528).

External	"	"	(529).

MUSCLES OF LEG (Fig. 330).

Tibialis anticus (521).

Extensor proprius hallucis (521).

Extensor longus digitorum (521).

Peroneus tertius (522).

MUSCLES OF DORSUM OF FOOT:

Extensor brevis digitorum (530).

ARTERIES (Fig. 378).
    Anterior tibial (641).
        Posterior recurrent (642).
        Superior fibular (642).
        Anterior recurrent (642).
        Muscular (642).
        Internal malleolar (643).
        External " (643).
    Dorsalis pedis (643).
        Tarsal (644).
        Metatarsal (644).
        Dorsalis hallucis (644).
        Communicating (644).
VEINS accompany the arteries.
NERVES:
    External popliteal (864).
    Anterior tibial (865) (Fig. 467).
        Branches (865).
    Musculo-cutaneous (865) (Fig. 467).
        Branches (865).

Fibular or Peroneal Region.
    Dissection (527):
    External annular ligament.
MUSCLES:
    Peroneus longus (527).
    Peroneus brevis (527).
NERVES:
    Musculo-cutaneous (865).
ARTERIES:
    Peroneal (646) (Fig. 377).

Posterior Tibio-Fibular Region.
    Dissection (522):
SUPERFICIAL VEINS (Fig. 392).
SUPERFICIAL NERVES (Figs. 509–510).
    External saphenous (863).
    Communicans peronei (865).

MUSCLES:
 Superficial layer.
  Gastrocnemius (522).
  Soleus (523).
  Plantaris (524).
  Tendo Achillis (523).
 Deep layer. *Dissection* (524).
  Deep fascia (524).
  Popliteus (524).
  Flexor longus hallucis (525).
  Flexor longus digitorum (525)..
  Tibialis posticus (526).
ARTERIES (Fig. 377).
 Popliteal.
  Posterior tibial (644).
  Peroneal (646).
  Muscular (647).
  Nutrient (647).
  Communicating (647).
  Internal calcanean (647).
NERVES (Fig. 510):
 Posterior tibial and branches (863)..
VEINS. Veins accompany the arteries.
Sole of the Foot.
 Dissection (529–530).
 Plantar fascia (529).
 MUSCLES: Three groups (530).
  First layer (Fig. 333).
   Abductor hallucis (530).
   Flexor brevis digitorum (530)..
   Abductor minimi digiti (531)..
   Fibrous sheaths (531).
  Second layer (Fig. 334).
   Flexor accessorius (532).
   Lumbricales (532).
  Third layer (Fig. 335).
   Flexor brevis hallucis (532)..

4

Knee-joint.
> Ligaments.
>> External (368–9).
>> Internal (369–0–1).
>> Synovial membrane (371).
>> Structures (372).
>> Blood supply (372).
>> Nerve supply (372).
>> Actions (372).
>> Surface form and surgical anatomy (374).

Articulations between tibia and fibula.
> Superior (376) ⎫
> Middle   (376) ⎬ ligaments.
> Inferior (377) ⎭
> Synovial membranes.
> Actions (377).

Ankle-joint (377).
> Ligaments (377–8).
> Synovial membrane (379).
> Relations (379).
> Blood supply (379).
> Nerve supply (379).
> Surface form (379).
> Surgical anatomy (379).

Tarsus.
> *Get a general idea of the articulations and ligaments of the tarsus* (Figs. 264–266).
> Blood supply.
> Nerve supply.

Tarso-metatarsal articulation (384–5).

Articulation of tarsal bones with each other (385).

Synovial membranes (385).

Nerve supply (386).

Metatarso-phalangeal articulations.
> Ligaments (386).

Articulations of phalanges.
> Ligaments (387).

PUBLICATIONS
OF

GEORGE WAHR,

Publisher and Bookseller,

ANN ARBOR, MICH.

———

A Text-Book of Elementary Mechanical Drawing for use in Office
or School.—By Clarence G. Wrentmore, B. S., C. E., and Her-
bert J. Goulding, B. S., M. E., *Instructors in Descriptive Geometry and Drawing* at the University of Michigan. Quarto,
109 pages, $1.00.

Plain Alphabets for Office and School.--Selected by C. G. Wrentmore, B. S., C. E., *Instructor in Descriptive Geometry and
Drawing*, University of Michigan. Pamphlet, 50 cents.

Tables for the Calculation of Simple or Compound Interest and Dis-
count and the Averaging of Accounts. The Values of Annuities,
Leases, Interest in Estates and the Accumulations and Values
of Investments at Simple or Compound Interest for all Rates and
Periods, also Tables for the Conversion of Securities and the
Value of Stocks and Bonds. With full Explanation for Use.—
By James C. Watson, Ph. D., LL. D. Quarto. Cloth, $2.50.

A Handbook of Practical Astronomy for University Students and
Engineers.—By W. W. Campbell, Sometime Instructor in the
University of Michigan, *Astronomer* in the Lick Observatory.
12 mo. 166 pages. $1.25.

The Theory of Substitutions and its Application to Algebra.—By
Dr. Eugene Netto, *Professor of Mathematics* in the University
of Giessen. Revised by the author and translated with his
permission, by F. N. Cole, Ph. D., formerly Assistant Professor
of Mathematics in the University of Michigan, *Professor of
Mathematics* in Columbia University. 8 vo. 301 pages.
Cloth, $3.00.

Mathematical Theories of Planetary Motions.—By Dr. Otto Dzio-
bek, *Privatdocent in the Royal Technical High School of Ber
lin, Charlottenburg.* Translated by Mark W. Harrington-
formerly Chief of the United States Weather Bureau, and,
Professor of Astronomy and Director of the Observatory at
the University of Michigan, President of the University of
Washington, and Wm. J. Hussey, *Assistant Professor of Astronomy* in the Leland Stanford, Junior, University. 8 vo. 294
pages. $3.50.

A French Reader for Beginners, with Notes and Vocabulary.—By
Moritz Levi, *Assistant Professor of French*, University of
Michigan, and Victor E. Francois, *Instructor in French*, Uni-
versity of Michigan. 12 mo. 261 pages. $1.00.

Les Aventures Du Dernier Abencerage Par Chateaubriand, Edited
with Notes and Vocabulary.—By Victor E. Francois, *Instructor in French* in the University of Michigan. Pamphlet, 35c.

Brief Outlines in European History. A Syllabus for the Use of Students in the University of Michigan.—By Earl Wilbur Dow.
Two parts each. 41 pages. Pamphlet, 35 cents.

The Study of Ethics. A Syllabus.—By John Dewey, *Professor of Philosophy* in the University of Chicago. Octavo. 144 pages. Cloth, $1.25.

Practical Pathology for Students and Physicians. A Manual of Laboratory and Post-Mortem Technic, Designed Especially for the Use of Junior and Senior Students in Pathology at the University of Michigan.—By Aldred Scott Warthin, Ph. D., M. D. *Instructor in Pathology*, University of Michigan. Octavo. 234 pages. Cloth, $1.50.

Directions for Work in the Histological Laboratory.—By G. Carl Huber, M. D., *Assistant Professor of Histology and Embryology*, University of Michigan. Second edition, revised and enlarged. Octavo. 191 pages. Cloth, $1.50.

Directions for Laboratory Work in Bacteriology.—By Frederick G. Novy, Sc. D., M. D., *Junior Professor of Hygiene and Physiological Chemistry*, University of Michigan. Octavo. 209 pages. Cloth, $1.50.

Directions for Laboratory Work in Urine Analysis.—By Frederick G. Novy, Sc D., M. D., *Junior Professor of Hygiene and Physiological Chemistry*, University of Michigan. Octavo. 102 pages. Cloth, $1.35.

Directions for Laboratory Work in Physiology for the Use of Medical Classes.—By W. H. Howell, Ph. D., M. D., *Professor of Physiology and Histology*. Pamphlet, 62 pages, 65 cents.

Select Methods in Inorganic Quantitative Analysis.—By Byron W. Cheever, A. M., M. D. Revised and enlarged by Frank Clemes Smith. Third edition. 12 mo. $1.75.

Syllabus of Lectures on Pharmacology and Therapeutics in the University of Michigan. Arranged Especially for the Use of the Classes Taking the Work in Pharmacology and Therapeutics at the University of Michigan.—By S. A. Matthews, M. D., *Assistant in Pharmacy and Therapeutics*, University of Michigan. 12 mo., 114 pages. $1.50.

Algebra—By Elmer A. Lyman, A. B., Edwin C. Goddard, Ph. B., and Arthur G. Hall, B. S., *Instructors in Mathematics*, University of Michigan. Octavo. 75 pages. Cloth, 90 cents.

Laboratory Manual of Elementary Chemistry.—By Jabez Montgomery, Ph. D., *Professor of Natural Science* in the Ann Arbor High School, and Roy B. Smith, *Assistant Professor in Chemical Laboratory*, Ann Arbor High School. 12 mo. 150 pages. Cloth, $1.00.

The Cranial Nerves. 12 pairs. By C. L. Ford, M. D., *Late Proffessor of Anatomy and Physiology* in University of Michigan. (Chart) 25 cents.

Classification of the Most Important Muscles of the Human Body, With Origin Insertion, Nervous Supply and Principal Action of Each.—By C. L. Ford, M. D., *Late Professor of Anatomy and Physiology* in the University of Michigan. Chart 50 cents.

Cronological Outline of Roman Literature.—By C. L. Meader, A. B., *Instructor in Latin* in University of Michigan. (Chart) 25 cents.

Outline of Anatomy. A Guide to the Dissection of the Human Body, Based on Gray's Anatomy.—54 pages. Boards. 60 cents.

Any of the above named books sent (post paid) on receipt of price.

GEORGE WAHR, Publisher and Bookseller, Ann Arbor, Mich.

www.ingramcontent.com/pod-product-compliance
Lightning Source LLC
Chambersburg PA
CBHW022013190326
41519CB00010B/1508